On Corpulence
By William Banting

© 2018 Phaistos Publishers

CORPULENCE.

Of all the parasites that affect humanity I do not know of, nor can I imagine any more distressing than that of Obesity, and having just emerged from a very long probation in this affliction, I am desirous of circulating my humble knowledge and experience for the benefit of my fellow man, with an earnest hope it may lead to the same comfort and happiness I now feel under the extraordinary change—which might almost be termed miraculous had it not been accomplished by the most simple common sense means.

Obesity seems to me very little understood or properly appreciated by the faculty and the public generally, or the former would long ere this have hit upon the cause for so lamentable a disease, and applied effective remedies, whilst the latter would have spared their injudicious indulgence in remarks and sneers, frequently painful in society, and which, even on the strongest mind, have an unhappy tendency; but I sincerely trust this humble effort at exposition may lead to a more perfect ventilation of the subject and a better feeling for the afflicted.

It would afford me infinite pleasure and satisfaction to name the author of my redemption from this calamity, as he is the only one that I have been able to find (and my search has not been sparing) who seems thoroughly up in the question; but such publicity might be construed improperly, and I have, therefore, only to offer my personal experience as to the stepping-stone to public investigation, and to proceed with my narrative of facts, earnestly hoping the reader will patiently peruse and thoughtfully consider it, with forbearance for any fault of style or diction, and for any seeming presumption in publishing it.

I have felt some difficulty in deciding on the proper and best course of action. At one time I thought the Editor of the Lancet would kindly publish a letter from me on the subject, but further reflection led me to doubt whether an insignificant individual would be noticed without some special introduction. In the April number of the Cornhill Magazine I read with much interest an article on the subject—defining tolerably well the effects, but offering no tangible remedy, or even positive solution of the problem—"What is the Cause of Obesity?" I was pleased with the article as a whole, but objected to some portions, and had prepared a letter to the Editor of that Magazine offering my experience on the subject, but it again struck me that an unknown individual like myself would have but little prospect of notice; so I finally resolved to publish and circulate this Pamphlet, with no other reason, motive, or expectation than an earnest desire to help those who happen to be afflicted as I was, for that corpulence is remediable I am well convinced, and shall be delighted if I can induce others to think so. The object I have in view impels me to enter into minute particulars as well as general observations, and to revert to bygone years, in order to show that I have spared no pains nor expense to accomplish the great end of stopping and curing obesity.

I am now nearly 66 years of age, about 5 feet 5 inches in stature, and, in August last (1862), weighed 202 lbs., which I think it right to name, because the article in the Cornhill Magazine presumes that a certain stature and age should bear, ordinarily, a certain weight, and I am quite of that opinion. I now weigh 167 lbs., showing a diminution of something like 1 lb. per week since August, and having now very nearly attained the happy medium, I have perfect confidence that a few more weeks will fully accomplish the object for which I have labored for the last thirty years, in vain, until it pleased Almighty Providence to direct me into the right and proper channel—the "tram-way," so to speak—of happy, comfortable existence.

Few men have led a more active life—bodily or mentally—from a constitutional anxiety for regularity, precision, and order, during fifty years' business career, from which I have now retired, so that my corpulence and subsequent obesity was not through neglect of necessary bodily activity, nor from excessive eating, drinking, or self-indulgence of any kind, except that I partook of the simple aliments of bread, milk, butter, beer, sugar, and potatoes more freely than my aged nature required, and hence, as I believe, the generation of the parasite, detrimental to comfort if not really to health.

I will not presume to descant on the bodily structural tissues, so fully canvassed in the Cornhill Magazine, nor how they are supported and renovated, having no mind or power to enter into these questions, which properly belong to the wise heads of the Faculty. None of my family on the side of either parent had any tendency to corpulence, and from my earliest years I had an inexpressible dread of such a calamity, so, when I was between thirty and forty years of age, finding a tendency to it creeping upon me, I consulted an eminent surgeon, now long deceased—a kind personal friend—who recommended increased bodily exertion before my ordinary daily labors began, and thought rowing an excellent plan. I had the command of a good, heavy, safe boat, lived near the river, and adopted it for a couple of hours in the early morning. It is true I gained muscular vigor, but with it a prodigious appetite, which I was compelled to indulge, and consequently increased in weight, until my kind old friend advised me to forsake the exercise.

He soon afterwards died, and, as the tendency to corpulence remained, I consulted other high orthodox authorities (never any inferior adviser), but all in vain. I have tried sea air and bathing in various localities, with much walking exercise; taken gallons of physic and liquor potasssæ, advisedly and abundantly; riding on horseback; the waters and climate of Leamington many times, as well as those of Cheltenham and Harrogate frequently; have lived upon sixpence a day, so to speak, and earned it, if bodily labor may be so construed; and have spared no trouble nor expense in consultations with the best authorities in the land, giving each and all a fair time for experiment, without any permanent remedy, as the evil still gradually increased.

I am under obligations to most of those advisers for the pains and interest they took in my case; but only to one for an effectual remedy.

When a corpulent man eats, drinks and sleeps well, has no pain to complain of and no particular organic disease, the judgment of able men seems paralyzed,— for I have been generally informed that corpulence is one of the natural results of increasing years; indeed one of the ablest authorities as a physician in the land told me he had gained 1 lb. in weight every year since he attained manhood, and was not surprised at my condition, but advised more bodily exercise—vapor-baths, and shampooing, in addition to the medicine given. Yet the evil still increased, and, like the parasite of barnacles on a ship, if it did not destroy the structure it obstructed its fair, comfortable progress in the path of life.

I have been in dock, perhaps, twenty times in as many years, for the reduction of this disease, and with little good effect—none lasting. Any one so afflicted is often subject to public remark, and though in conscience he may care little about it, I am confident no man laboring under obesity can be quite insensible to the sneers and remarks of the cruel and injudicious in public assemblies, public vehicles, or the ordinary street traffic; nor to the annoyance of finding no adequate space in a public assembly if he should seek amusement or need refreshment, and therefore he naturally keeps away as much as possible from places where he is likely to be made the object of the taunts and remarks of others. I am as regardless of public remark as most men, but I have felt these difficulties and therefore avoided such circumscribed accommodation and notice, and by that means have been deprived of many advantages to health and comfort.

Although no very great size or weight, still I could not stoop to tie my shoe, so to speak, nor attend to the little offices humanity requires without considerable pain and difficulty, which only the corpulent can understand; I have been compelled to go down stairs slowly backwards, to save the jar of increased weight upon the ankle and knee joints, and been obliged to puff and blow with every slight exertion, particularly that of going up stairs. I have spared no pains to remedy this by low living (moderation and light food was generally prescribed, but I had no direct bill of fare to know what was really intended), and that, consequently, brought the system into a low impoverished state, without decreasing corpulence, caused many obnoxious boils, to appear, and two rather formidable carbuncles, for which I was ably operated upon and fed into increased obesity.

At this juncture (about three years back) Turkish baths became the fashion, and I was advised to adopt them as a remedy. With the first few I found immense benefit in power and elasticity for walking exercise; so, believing I had found the "philosopher's stone," pursued them three times a week till I had taken fifty, then less frequently (as I began to fancy, with some reason, that so many weakened my constitution) till I had taken ninety, but never succeeded in losing more than 6 lbs. weight during the whole course, and I gave up the plan as worthless; though I have full belief in their cleansing properties, and their value in colds, rheumatism, and many other ailments.

I then fancied increased obesity materially affected a slight umbilical rupture, if it did not cause it, and that another bodily ailment to which I had been subject was also augmented. This led me to other medical advisers, to whom I am also indebted for much kind consideration, though, unfortunately, they failed in relieving me. At last, finding my sight failing and my hearing greatly impaired, I consulted, in August last, an eminent aural surgeon, who made light of the case, looked into my ears, sponged them internally, and blistered the outside, without the slightest benefit, neither inquiring into any of my bodily ailments, which he probably thought unnecessary, nor affording me even time to name them.

I was not at all satisfied, but on the contrary was in a worse plight than when I went to him; however, he soon after left town for his annual holiday, which proved the greatest possible blessing to me, because it compelled me to seek other assistance, and happily, I found the right man, who unhesitatingly said he believed my ailments were caused principally by corpulence, and prescribed a certain diet—no medicine, beyond a morning cordial as a corrective—with immense effect and advantage both to my hearing and the decrease ot my corpulency.

For the sake of argument and illustration I will presume that certain articles of ordinary diet, however beneficial in youth, are prejudicial in advanced life, like beans to a horse, whose common, ordinary food is hay and corn. It may be useful food occasionally, under peculiar circumstances, but detrimental as a constancy. I will, therefore, adopt the analogy, and call such food human beans. The items from which I was advised to abstain as much as possible were:—Bread, butter, milk, sugar, beer, and potatoes, which had been the main (and, I thought, innocent) elements of my existence, or, at all events, they had for many years been adopted freely. These, said my excellent adviser, contain starch and saccharine matter, tending to create fat, and should be avoided altogether. At the first blush it seemed to me that I had little left to live upon, but my kind friend soon showed me there was ample, and I was only too happy to give the plan a fair trial, and, within a very few days, found immense benefit from it. It may better elucidate the dietary plan if I describe generally what I have sanction to take, and that man must be an extraordinary person who would desire a better table:—

For breakfast, I take four or five ounces of beef, mutton, kidneys, broiled fish, bacon, or cold meat of any kind except pork; a large cup of tea (without milk or sugar), a little biscuit, or one ounce of dry toast.

For dinner, five or six ounces of any fish except salmon, any meat except pork, any vegetable except potato, one ounce of dry toast, fruit out of a pudding, any kind of poultry or game, and two or three glasses of good claret, sherry, or Madeira—champagne, port and beer forbidden.

For tea, two or three ounces of fruit, a rusk or two, and a cup of tea without milk or sugar.

For supper, three or four ounces of meat or fish, similar to dinner, with a glass or two of claret.

For nightcap, if required, a tumbler of grog—(gin, whiskey, or brandy, without sugar)—or a glass or two of claret or sherry.

This plan leads to an excellent night's rest, with from six to eight hours' sound sleep. The dry toast or rusk may have a table spoonful of spirit to soften it, which will prove acceptable. Perhaps I did not wholly escape starchy or saccharine matter, but scrupulously avoided those beans, such as milk, sugar, beer, butter, &c., which were known to contain them.

On rising in the morning I take a table spoonful of a special corrective cordial, which may be called the Balm of Life, in a wine-glass of water, a most grateful draught, as it seems to carry away all the dregs left in the stomach after digestion, but is not aperient; then I take 5 or 6 ounces of solid and 8 of liquid for breakfast; 8 ounces of solid and 8 of liquid for dinner; 3 ounces of solid and 8 of liquid for tea; 4 ounces of solid and 6 of liquid for supper, and the grog afterwards, if I please. I am not, however, strictly limited to any quantity at either meal, so that the nature of the food is rigidly adhered to.

Experience has taught me to believe that these human beans are the most insidious enemies man, with a tendency to corpulence in advanced life, can possess, though eminently friendly to youth. He may very prudently mount guard against such an enemy if he is not a fool to himself, and I fervently hope this truthful unvarnished tale may lead him to make a trial of my plan, which I sincerely recommend to public notice—not with any ambitious motive, but in sincere good faith to help my fellow creatures to obtain the marvellous blessings I have found within the short period of a few months.

I do not recommend every corpulent man to rush headlong into such a change of diet (certainly not), but to act advisedly and after full consultation with a physician.

My former dietary table was bread and milk for breakfast, or a pint of tea with plenty of milk and sugar, and buttered toast; meat, beer, much bread (of which I was always very fond), and pastry for dinner, the meal of tea similar to that of breakfast, and generally a fruit tart or bread and milk for supper. I had little comfort and far less sound sleep.

It certainly appears to me that my present dietary table is far superior to the former—more luxurious and liberal, independent of its blessed effect—but when it is proved to be more healthful, comparisons are simply ridiculous, and I can hardly imagine any man, even in sound health, would choose the former, even if it were not an enemy; but, when it is shown to be, as in my case, inimical both to health and comfort, I can hardly conceive there is any man who would not willingly avoid it. I can conscientiously assert I never lived so well as under the new plan of dietary, which I should have formerly thought a dangerous, extravagant trespass upon health. I am very much better, bodily and mentally, and pleased to believe that I hold the reins of health and comfort in my own hands; and, though at sixty-five years of age, I cannot expect to remain free from some coming natural infirmity that all flesh is heir to, I cannot, at the present time, complain of one. It is simply miraculous, and I am thankful to Almighty Providence for directing me, through an extraordinary chance, to the care of a man who could work such a change in so short a time.

Oh! that the faculty would look deeper into and make themselves better acquainted with the crying evil of obesity—that dreadful tormenting parasite on health and comfort. Their fellow men might not descend into early premature graves, as I believe many do, from what is termed apoplexy, and certainly would not during their sojourn on earth, endure so much bodily and consequently mental infirmity.

Corpulence, though giving no actual pain, as it appears to me, must naturally press with undue violence upon the bodily viscera, driving one part upon another and stopping the free action of all. I am sure it did in my particular case, and the result of my experience is briefly as follows:

I have not felt so well as now for the last twenty years.

Have suffered no inconvenience whatever in the probational remedy.

Am reduced many inches in bulk, and 35 lbs. in weight in thirty-eight weeks.

Come down stairs forward naturally, with perfect ease.

Go up stairs and take ordinary exercise freely, without the slightest inconvenience.

Can perform every necessary office for myself.

The umbilical rupture is greatly ameliorated—and gives me no anxiety.

My sight is restored—my hearing improved.

My other bodily ailments are ameliorated—indeed almost past into matters of history.

I have placed a thank-offering of £50 in the hands of my kind medical adviser, for distribution amongst his favorite hospitals, after gladly paying his usual fees, and still remain under overwhelming obligations for his care and attention, which I can never hope to repay. Most thankful to Almighty Providence for mercies received, and determined to press the case into public notice as a token of gratitude.

I have the pleasure to afford, in conclusion, a satisfactory confirmation of my report, in stating that a corpulent friend of mine, who, like myself, is possessed of a generally sound constitution, was laboring under frequent palpitations of the heart and sensations of fainting, was, at my instigation, induced to place himself in the hands of my medical adviser, with the same gradual beneficial results. He is at present under the same ordeal, and in eight weeks has profited even more largely than I did in that short period; he has lost the palpitations, and is becoming, so to speak, a new made man—thankful to me for advising, and grateful to the eminent counsellor to whom I referred him—and he looks forward with good hope to a perfect cure.

I am fully persuaded that hundreds, if not thousands, of our fellow men might profit equally by a similar course; but, constitutions not being all alike, a different course of treatment may be advisable for the removal of so tormenting an affliction.

My kind and valued medical adviser is not a doctor for obesity, but stands on the pinnacle of fame in the treatment of another malady, which, as he well knows is frequently induced by the disease of which I am speaking, and I sincerely trust most of my corpulent friends (and there are thousands of corpulent people whom I dare not so rank) may be led into my tram-road. To any such I am prepared to offer the further key of knowledge by naming the man. It might seem invidious to do so now, but I shall only be too happy, if applied to by letter in good faith, or if any doubt should exist as to the correctness of this statement.

WILLIAM BANTING, Sen.,

Late of No. 27, St. James St., Piccadilly,

Now of No. 4, The Terrace, Kensington.

May, 1863.

ADDENDA.

Having exhausted the first edition (1000 copies) of the foregoing pamphlet; and a period of one year having elapsed since commencing the admirable course of diet which has led to such inestimable beneficial results, and, "as I expected and desired," having quite succeeded in attaining the happy medium of weight and bulk I had so long ineffectually sought, which appears necessary to health at my age and stature—I feel impelled, by a sense of public duty, to offer the results of my experience in a second edition. It has been suggested that I should have sold the pamphlet, devoting any profit to charity as more agreeable and useful; and I had intended to adopt such a course, but on reflection feared my motives might be mistaken; I therefore respectfully present this (like the first Edition) to the public gratuitously, earnestly hoping the subject may be taken up by medical men and thoroughly ventilated.

It may (and I hope will) be as satisfactory to the public to hear as it is for me to state, that the first edition has been attended with very comforting results to other sufferers from corpulence, as the remedial system therein described was to me under that terrible disease, which was my main object in publishing my convictions on the subject. It has moreover attained a success, produced flattering compliments, and an amount of attention I could hardly have imagined possible. The pleasure and satisfaction this has afforded me, is ample compensation for the trouble and expense I have incurred, and I most sincerely trust, "as I verily believe," this second edition will be accompanied by similar satisfactory results from a more extensive circulation. If so, it will inspirit me to circulate further editions, whilst a corpulent person exists, requiring, as I think, this system of diet, or so long as my motives cannot be mistaken, and are thankfully appreciated.

My weight is reduced 46 lbs., and as the very gradual reductions which I am able to show may be interesting to many, I have great pleasure in stating them, believing they serve to demonstrate further the merit of the system pursued.

My weight on 26th of August, 1862, was 202 lbs.

		lbs.		lbs.	
On	7th September,	it was 200,	having lost 2		
	27th " "	197	"	3	more.
	19th October	" 193	"	4	"
	9th November	" 190	"	3	"
	3rd December	" 187	"	3	"
	24th " "	184	"	3	"
	14th Jan., 1863	" 182	"	2	"
	4th February	" 180	"	2	"
	25th " "	178	"	2	"
	18th March "	176	"	2	"
	8th April "	173	"	3	"
	29th " "	170	"	3	"
	20th May "	167	"	3	"
	10th June "	164	"	3	"
	1st July "	161	"	3	"
	22d July "	159	"	2	"
	12th August "	157	"	2	"
	26th " "	156	"	1	"

12th September	"	156	"	0	"

Total loss of weight   46   lbs.

My girth is reduced round the waist, in tailor phraseology, 12¼ inches, which extent was hardly conceivable even by my friends, or my respected medical adviser, until I put on my former clothing, over what I now wear, which was a thoroughly convincing proof of the remarkable change. These important desiderata have been attained by the most easy and comfortable means, with but little medicine, and almost entirely by a system of diet that formerly I should have thought dangerously generous. I am told by all who know me that my personal appearance is greatly improved, and that I seem to bear the stamp of good health; this may be a matter of opinion or friendly remark, but I can honestly assert that I feel restored in health, "bodily and mentally," appear to have more muscular power and vigor, eat and drink with a good appetite, and sleep well. All symptoms of acidity, indigestion and heartburn (with which I was frequently tormented) have vanished. I have left off using boot hooks, and other such aids, which were indispensable, but being now able to stoop with ease and freedom, are unnecessary. I have lost the feeling of occasional faintness, and what I think a remarkable blessing and comfort is, that I have been able safely to leave off knee bandages, which I had worn necessarily for 20 past years, and given up a truss almost entirely; indeed, I believe I might wholly discard it with safety, but am advised to wear it at least occasionally for the present.

Since publishing my pamphlet, I have felt constrained to send a copy of it to my former medical advisers, and to ascertain their opinions on the subject. They did not dispute or question the propriety of the system, but either dared not venture its practice upon a man of my age, or thought it too great a sacrifice of personal comfort to be generally advised or adopted, and I fancy neither of them appeared to feel the fact of the misery of corpulence. One eminent physician, as I before stated, assured me that increasing weight was a necessary result of advancing years; another, equally eminent, to whom I had been directed by a very friendly third, who had most kindly but ineffectually failed in a remedy, added to my weight in a few weeks instead of abating the evil. These facts lead me to believe the question is not sufficiently observed or even regarded.

The great charm and comfort of the system is, that its effects are palpable within a week of trial, which creates a natural stimulus to persevere for a few weeks more, when the fact becomes established beyond question.

I only entreat all persons suffering from corpulence to make a fair trial for just one clear month, as I am well convinced they will afterwards pursue a course which yields such extraordinary benefit, till entirely and effectually relieved, and be it remembered, by the sacrifice merely of simple, for the advantage of more generous and comforting food. The simple dietary evidently adds fuel to the fire, whereas the superior and liberal seems to extinguish it.

I am delighted to be able to assert that I have proved the great merit and advantage of the system by its result in several other cases, similar to my own, and have full confidence that within the next twelve months I shall know of many more cases restored from the disease of corpulence, for I have received the kindest possible letters from many afflicted strangers and friends, as well as similar personal observations from others, whom I have converse with, and assurances from most of them that they will kindly inform me the result for my own private satisfaction. Many are practicing the diet after consultation with their own medical advisers; some few have gone to mine, and others are practicing upon their own convictions of the advantages detailed in the pamphlet, though I recommend all to act advisedly, in case their constitutions should differ. I am, however, so perfectly satisfied of the great unerring benefits of this system of diet, that I shall spare no trouble to circulate my humble experience. The amount and character of my correspondence on the subject has been strange and singular, but most satisfactory to my mind and feelings.

I am now in that happy, comfortable state that I should not hesitate to indulge in any fancy in regard to diet, but if I did so should watch the consequences, and not continue any course which might add to weight or bulk and consequent discomfort.

Is not the system suggestive to artists and men of sedentary employment who cannot spare time for exercise, consequently become corpulent, and clog the little muscular action with a superabundance of fat, thus easily avoided?

Pure, genuine bread, may be the staff of life, as it is termed. It is so, particularly in youth, but I feel certain it is more wholesome in advanced life if thoroughly toasted, as I take it. My impression is that any starchy or saccharine matter tends to the disease of corpulence in advanced life, and whether it be swallowed in that form or generated in the stomach, that all things tending to these elements should be avoided, of course always under sound medical authority.

WILLIAM BANTING.

CONCLUDING ADDENDA.

It is very satisfactory to me to be able to state, that I remained at the same standard of bulk and weight for several weeks after the 26th August, when I attained the happy natural medium, since which time I have varied in weight from two to three pounds, more or less. I have seldom taken the morning draught since that time, and have frequently indulged my fancy, experimentally, in using milk, sugar, butter, and potatoes—indeed, I may say all the forbidden articles except beer, in moderation, with impunity, but always as an exception, not as a rule. This deviation, however, convinces me that I hold the power of maintaining the happy medium in my own hands.

A kind friend has lately furnished me with a tabular statement in regard to weight as proportioned to stature, which, under present circumstances and the new movement, may be interesting and useful to corpulent readers:

STATURE.	WEIGHT.	
5 ft. 1	should be 8 stone 8	or 120 lbs.
5 " 2	" 9" 0 " 126	"
5 " 3	" 9" 7 " 133	"
5 " 4	" 9" 10 " 136	"
5 " 5	" 10" 2 " 142	"
5 " 6	" 10" 5 " 145	"
5 " 7	" 10" 8 " 148	"
5 " 8	" 11" 1 " 155	"
5 " 9	" 11" 8 " 162	"
5 " 10	" 12" 1 " 169	"
5 " 11	" 12" 6 " 174	"
6 " 0	" 12" 10 " 178	"

This tabular statement, taken from a mean average of 2,648 healthy men, was formed and arranged for an Insurance Company by the late Dr. John Hutchinson. It answered as a pretty good standard, and insurances were regulated upon it. His calculations were made upon the volume of air passing in and out of the lungs, and this was his guide as to how far the various organs of the body were in health, and the lungs in particular. It may be viewed as some sort of probable rule, yet only as an average—some in health weighing more by many pounds than others. It must not be looked upon as infallible, but only as a sort of general reasonable guide to Nature's great and mighty work.

On a general view of the question I think it may be conceded that a frame of low stature was hardly intended to bear heavy weight. Judging from this tabular statement I ought to be considerably lighter than I am at present: I shall not, however, covet or aim at such a result, nor, on the other hand feel alarmed if I decrease a little more in weight and bulk.

I am certainly more sensitive to cold since I have lost the superabundant fat, but this is remedial by another garment, far more agreeable and satisfactory. Many of my friends have said, "Oh! you have done well so far, but take care you don't go too far!" I fancy such a circumstance, with such a dietary, very unlikely, if not impossible; but feeling that I have now nearly attained the right standard of bulk and weight proportional to my stature and age (between 10 and 11 stone), I should not hesitate to partake of a fattening dietary occasionally, to preserve the happy standard, if necessary; indeed, I am allowed to do so by my medical adviser, but I shall always observe a careful watch upon myself to discover the effect, and act accordingly, so that, if I choose to spend a day or two with Dives, so to speak, I must not forget to devote the next to Lazarus.

The remedy may be as old as the hills, as I have since been told, but its application is of very recent date; and it astonishes me that such a light should have remained so long unnoticed and hidden, as not to afford a glimmer to my anxious mind in a search for it during the last twenty years, even in directions where it might have been expected to be known. I would rather presume it is a new light, than that it was purposely hidden merely because the disease of obesity was not immediately dangerous to existence, nor thought to be worthy of serious consideration. Little do the faculty imagine the misery and bitterness to life through the parasite of corpulence or obesity.

I can now confidently say that quantity of diet may be safely left to the natural appetite; and that it is the quality only, which is essential to abate and cure corpulence. I stated the quantities of my own dietary, because it was part of a truthful report, but some correspondents have doubted whether it should be more or less in their own cases, a doubt which would be better solved by their own appetite, or medical adviser. I have heard a graphic remark by a corpulent man, which may not be inappropriately stated here, that big houses were not formed with scanty materials. This, however, is a poor excuse for self indulgence in improper food, or for not consulting medical authority.

The approach of corpulence is so gradual that, until it is far advanced, persons rarely become objects of attention. Many have even congratulated themselves on their comely appearance, and have not sought advice or a remedy for what they did not consider an evil, for an evil I can say most truly it is, when in much excess, to which point it must, in my opinion arrive, unless obviated by proper means.

Many have wished to know (as future readers may) the nature of the morning draught, or where it could be obtained, but believing it would have been highly imprudent on my part to have presumed that what was proper for my constitution was applicable to all indiscriminately, I could only refer them to a medical adviser for any aid beyond the dietary; assuring them, however, it was not a dram but of an alkaline character.

Some, I believe, would willingly submit to even a violent remedy, so that an immediate benefit could be produced; this is not the object of the treatment, as it cannot but be dangerous, in my humble opinion, to reduce a disease of this nature suddenly; they are probably then too prone to despair of success, and consider it as unalterably connected with their constitution. Many under this feeling doubtless return to their former habits, encouraged so to act by the ill-judged advice of friends, who, I am persuaded (from the correspondence I have had on this most interesting subject) become unthinking accomplices in the destruction of those whom they regard and esteem.

The question of four meals a-day, and the night cap, has been abundantly and amusingly criticized. I ought perhaps to have stated as an excuse for such liberality of diet, that I breakfast between eight and nine o'clock, dine between one and two, take my slight tea meal between five and six, sup at nine, and only take the night cap when inclination directs. My object in naming it at all was, that, as a part of a whole system, it should be known, and to show it is not forbidden to those who are advised that they need such a luxury; nor was it injurious in my case. Some have inquired whether smoking was prohibited. It was not.

It has also been remarked that such a dietary as mine was too good and expensive for a poor man, and that I had wholly lost sight of that class; but a very poor corpulent man is not so frequently met with, inasmuch as the poor cannot afford the simple inexpensive means for creating fat; but when the tendency does exist in that class, I have no doubt it can be remedied by abstinence from the forbidden articles, and a moderate indulgence in such cheap stimulants as may be recommended by a medical adviser, whom they have ample chances of consulting gratuitously.

I have a very strong feeling that gout (another terrible parasite upon humanity) might be greatly relieved, if not cured entirely, by this proper natural dietary, and sincerely hope some person so afflicted may be induced to practice the harmless plan for three months (as I certainly would if the case were my own) to prove it; but not without advice.

My impression from the experiments I have tried on myself of late is, that saccharine matter is the great moving cause of fatty corpulence. I know that it produces in my individual case increased weight and a large amount of flatulence, and believe, that not only sugar, but all elements tending to create saccharine matter in the process of digestion, should be avoided. I apprehend it will be found in bread, butter, milk, beer, port wine, and champagne; I have not found starchy matter so troublesome as the saccharine, which, I think, largely increases acidity as well as fat, but, with ordinary care and observation, people will soon find what food rests easiest in the stomach, and avoid that which does not, during the probationary trial of the proposed dietary. Vegetables and ripe or stewed fruit I have found ample aperients. Failing this, medical advice should be sought.

The word "parasite" has been much commented upon, as inappropriate to any but a living creeping thing (of course I use the word in a figurative sense, as a burden to the flesh), but if fat is not an insidious creeping enemy, I do not know what is. I should have equally applied the word to gout, rheumatism, dropsy, and many other diseases.

Whereas hitherto the appeals to me to know the name of my medical adviser have been very numerous, I may say hundreds, which I have gladly answered, though forming no small item of the expense incurred, and whereas the very extensive circulation expected of the third edition is likely to lead to some thousands of similar applications, I feel bound in self-defence, to state that the medical gentleman to whom I am so deeply indebted is Mr. Harvey, Soho Square, London, whom I consulted for deafness. In the first and second editions, I thought that to give his name would appear like a puff, which I know he abhors; indeed, I should prefer not to do so now, but cannot in justice to myself, incur further probable expense (which I fancy inevitable) besides the personal trouble, for which I cannot afford time, and, therefore, feel no hesitation to refer to him as my guarantee for the truth of the pamphlet.

One material point I should be glad to impress on my corpulent readers—it is, to get accurately weighed at starting upon the fresh system, and continue to do so weekly or monthly, for the change will be so truly palpable by this course of examination, that it will arm them with perfect confidence in the merit and ultimate success of the plan. I deeply regret not having secured a photographic portrait of my original figure in 1862, to place in juxta position with one of my present form. It might have amused some, but certainly would have been very convincing to others, and astonishing to all that such an effect should have been so readily and speedily produced by the simple natural cause of exchanging a meagre for a generous dietary under proper advice.

I shall ever esteem it a great favor if persons relieved and cured, as I have been, will kindly let me know of it; the information will be truly gratifying to my mind. That the system is a great success, I have not a shadow of doubt from the numerous reports sent with thanks by strangers as well as from friends from all parts of the kingdom; and I am truly thankful to have been the humble instrument of disseminating the blessing and experience I have attained through able counsel and natural causes by proper perseverance.

I have now finished my task, and trust my humble efforts may prove to be good seed well sown, that will fructify and produce a large harvest of benefit to my fellow creatures. I also hope the faculty generally may be led more extensively to ventilate this question of corpulence or obesity, so that, instead of one, two, or three able practitioners, there may be as many hundreds distributed in the various parts of the United Kingdom. In such case, I am persuaded, that those diseases, like Reverence and Golden Pippins, will be very rare.

APPENDIX.

Since publishing the third edition of my pamphlet, I have earnestly pressed my medical adviser to explain the reasons for so remarkable a result as I and others have experienced from the dietary system he prescribed, and I hope he may find time to do so shortly, as I believe it would be highly interesting to the Faculty and the public generally. He has promised this at his leisure.

Numerous applications having been made to me on points to which I had not alluded, in which my correspondents felt some doubt and interest, I take this opportunity of making some few corrections in my published dietary:—

I ought, "it seems," to have excepted veal, owing to its indigestible quality, as well as pork for its fattening character; also herrings and eels (owing to their oily nature), being as injurious as salmon. In respect to vegetables, not only should potatoes be prohibited, but parsnips, beetroot, turnips, and carrots. The truth is, I seldom or ever partook of these objectionable articles myself, and did not reflect that others might do so, or that they were forbidden. Green vegetables are considered very beneficial, and I believe should be adopted at all times. I am indebted to the "Cornhill Magazine" and other journals for drawing my attention to these dietetic points. I can now also state that eggs, if not hard boiled, are unexceptionable, that cheese, if sparingly used, and plain boiled rice seem harmless.

Some doubts have been expressed in regard to the vanishing point of such a descending scale, but it is a remarkable fact that the great and most palpable diminution in weight and bulk occurs within the first forty-eight hours, the descent is then more gradual. My own experience, and that of others, assures me (if medical authority be first consulted as to the complaint) that with such slight extraneous aid as medicine can afford, nature will do her duty, and only her duty: firstly, by relieving herself of immediate pressure she will be enabled to move more freely in her own beautiful way, and secondly, by pursuing the same course to work speedy amelioration and final cure. The vanishing point is only when the disease is stopped and the parasite annihilated.

It may interest my readers to know that I have now apparently attained the standard natural at my age (10 stone 10, or 150 lbs.), as my weight now varies only to the extent of 1 lb., more or less in the course of a month. According to Dr. Hutchinson's tables I ought to lose still more, but cannot do so without resorting to medicine; and, feeling in sound vigorous health, I am perfectly content to wait upon nature for any further change.

In my humble judgment the dietary is the principal point in the treatment of Corpulence, and it appears to me, moreover, that if properly regulated it becomes in a certain sense a medicine. The system seems to me to attack only the superfluous deposit of fat, and, as my medical friend informs me, purges the blood, rendering it more pure and healthy, strengthens the muscles and bodily viscera, and I feel quite convinced sweetens life if it does not prolong it.

It is truly gratifying to me to be able now to add that many other of the most exalted members of the Faculty have honoured my movement in the question with their approbation.

I consider it a public duty further to state, that Mr. Harvey, whom I have named on the 24th page as my kind medical adviser in the cure of Corpulence, is not Dr. John Harvey, who has published a Pamphlet on Corpulence assimilating with some of the features and the general aspect of mine, and which has been considered (as I learn from correspondents who have obtained it) the work of my medical friend. It is not.

I am glad, therefore, to repeat that my medical adviser was, and is still, Mr. William Harvey, F.R.C.S., No. 2, Soho Square, London, W.

WILLIAM BANTING.

April, 1864.

MR. HARVEY'S REMARKS.

"My patient, Mr. Banting, having published for the benefit of his fellow sufferers, some account of the diet which I recommended him to adopt with a view to relieve him of a distressing degree of hypertrophy of the adipose tissue. I have been frequently urged by him to explain the principles upon which I was enabled to treat with success this inconvenient, and in some instances, distressing condition of the system.

"The simple history of my finding occasion to investigate this subject is as follows:—When in Paris, in the year 1856, I took the opportunity of attending a discussion on the views of M. Bernard, who was at that time propounding his now generally admitted theory of the liver functions. After he had discovered by chemical processes and physiological experiments, which it is unnecessary for me to recapitulate here, that the liver not only secreted bile, but also a peculiar amyloid or starch-like product which he called glucose, and which in its chemical and physical properties appeared to be nearly allied to saccharine matter, he further found that this glucose could be directly produced in the liver by the ingestion of sugar and its ally starch, and that in diabetes it existed there in considerable excess. It had long been well known that a purely animal diet greatly assisted in checking the secretion of diabetic urine; and it seemed to follow, as a matter of course, that the total abstinence from saccharine and farinaceous matter must drain the liver of this excessive amount of glucose, and thus arrest in a similar proportion the diabetic tendency. Reflecting on this chain of argument, and knowing too that a saccharine and farinaceous diet is used to fatten certain animals, and that in diabetes, the whole of the fat of the body rapidly disappears, it occurred to me that excessive obesity might be allied to diabetes as to its cause, although widely diverse in its development: and that if a purely animal diet was useful in the latter disease, a combination of animal food with such vegetable matters as contained neither sugar nor starch, might serve to arrest the undue formation of fat. I soon afterwards had an opportunity of testing this idea. A dispensary patient, who consulted me for deafness, and who was enormously corpulent, I found to have no distinguishable disease of the ear. I therefore suspected that his deafness arose from the great development of adipose matter in the throat, pressing upon and stopping up the eustachian tubes. I subjected him to a strict non-farinaceous and non-saccharine diet, and treated him with the volatile alkali alluded to in his Pamphlet, and occasional aperients, and in about seven months he was reduced to almost normal proportions, his hearing restored, and his general health immensely improved. This case seemed to give substance and reality to my conjectures, which further experience has confirmed.

"When we consider that fat is what is termed hydro carbon, and deposits itself so insidiously and yet so gradually amongst the tissues of the body, it is at once manifest that we require such substances as contain a superfluity of oxygen and nitrogen to arrest its formation and to vitalize the system. That is the principal upon which the diet suggested in his Pamphlet works, and explains on the one hand the necessity of abstaining from all vegetable roots which hold a large quantity of saccharine matter, and on the other the beneficial effects derivable from those vegetables, the fruits of which are on the exterior of the earth, as they lose, probably by means of the sun's action, a large proportion of their sugar.

"With regard to the tables of Dr. Hutchinson, referred to in his Pamphlet, it is no doubt difficult, as he says, to determine what is a man's proper weight, which must be influenced by various causes. Those tables, however, were formed by him on the principle of considering the amount of air which the lungs in their healthy state can receive and apply to the oxydation of the blood. I gave them to Mr. Banting as an indication only of what the approximate weight of adult persons in proportion to their stature should be, and with the view of proving to them the importance of keeping down the tendency to grow fat; for, as that tendency increases, the capacity of the lungs, and consequently the vitality and power of the whole system must diminish. In conclusion, I would suggest the propriety of advising a dietary such as this in diseases that are in any way influenced by a disordered condition of the hepatic functions, as they cannot fail to yield in some degree to this simple method of treatment if fairly and properly carried out; it remains for me to watch its progress in a more limited sphere.

"William Harvey, F.R.C.S.,

"Surgeon to the Royal Dispensary,

for Diseases of the Ear."

2, Soho Square,

April, 1864.